# BREATHING EASY: NOURISHING RECIPES FOR ASTHMA WELLNESS

## Asthma-Friendly Recipes Cookbook

LAUREN WILLS

# CONTENTS


CONTENTS ...................................................................3

INTRODUCTION ..................................................6

ASTHMA-FRIENDLY RECIPES ...............................8

Recipe 1: Grilled Chicken and Veggie Wrap .......................8

Recipe 2: Quinoa and Black Bean Salad ........................ 10

Recipe 3: Baked Salmon with Lemon-Dill Sauce .............11

Recipe 4: Spinach and Mushroom Stuffed Chicken Breast ................................................................ 13

Recipe 5: Lentil and Vegetable Soup ................................ 15

Recipe 6: Grilled Vegetable and Quinoa Bowl.................. 16

Recipe 7: Creamy Tomato Basil Soup .............................. 18

Recipe 8: Roasted Butternut Squash and Apple Salad.....20

Recipe 9: Sweet Potato and Black Bean Enchiladas......... 21

Recipe 10: Mediterranean Chickpea Salad ......................23

Recipe 11: Lemon Garlic Shrimp and Asparagus..............25

Recipe 12: Creamy Avocado and Spinach Pasta ..............26

Recipe 13: Turkey and Vegetable Stir-Fry ......................28

Recipe 14: Zucchini Noodles with Pesto and Cherry Tomatoes .......................................................................30

Recipe 15: Roasted Red Pepper Hummus ........................ 31

Recipe 16: Teriyaki Tofu and Vegetable Skewers ............. 33

Recipe 17: Eggplant and Tomato Stew ............................. 34

Recipe 18: Sweet and Spicy Glazed Salmon ..................... 36

Recipe 19: Vegan Lentil and Mushroom Shepherd's Pie .. 37

Recipe 20: Caprese Stuffed Portobello Mushrooms ......... 40

Recipe 21: Chickpea and Vegetable Curry ....................... 41

Recipe 22: Almond-Crusted Baked Chicken Tenders ...... 43

Recipe 23: Roasted Beet and Goat Cheese Salad ............. 45

Recipe 24: Spinach and Feta Stuffed Mushrooms ........... 47

Recipe 25: Blueberry and Almond Overnight Oats ......... 48

Recipe 26: Quinoa and Roasted Vegetable Bowl ............. 50

Recipe 27: Lemon Herb Baked Salmon ........................... 52

Recipe 28: Black Bean and Corn Salsa ............................ 53

Recipe 29: Cucumber and Dill Greek Yogurt Dip ............ 55

Recipe 30: Baked Sweet Potato Fries .............................. 56

Recipe 31: Ginger Turmeric Tea ...................................... 58

Recipe 32: Mediterranean Stuffed Bell Peppers .............. 59

Recipe 33: Coconut Banana Smoothie ............................. 61

Recipe 34: Tomato Basil Quinoa Salad ............................ 62

Recipe 35: Baked Cod with Lemon and Herbs ................ 63

Recipe 36: Mango and Spinach Salad with Citrus Dressing ................................................................. 65

Recipe 37: Lemon Herb Quinoa Salad.................... 66

Recipe 38: Roasted Brussels Sprouts with Balsamic Glaze ................................................................. 68

Recipe 39: Vegan Lentil Soup ............................... 69

Recipe 40: Grilled Shrimp and Pineapple Skewers........... 71

Recipe 41: Turkey and Vegetable Stir-Fry ...................... 73

Recipe 42: Berry and Spinach Smoothie Bowl ................ 75

Recipe 43: Turkey and Black Bean Chili.......................... 76

Recipe 44: Caprese Salad with Balsamic Reduction ........ 78

Recipe 45: Spaghetti Squash with Pesto ...........................80

Recipe 46: Greek Chicken Souvlaki ................................. 81

Recipe 47: Sweet Potato and Black Bean Tacos................ 83

Recipe 48: Mango and Avocado Salad.............................. 85

Recipe 49: Broccoli and Cheddar Stuffed Potatoes ..........86

Recipe 50: Teriyaki Salmon ..............................................88

CONCLUSION ................................................................ 91

# INTRODUCTION

Welcome to "Breathing Easy: Nourishing Recipes for Asthma Wellness," a cookbook specially crafted to enhance your culinary journey while prioritizing your respiratory health. We understand that managing asthma can be a daily challenge, and nutrition plays a pivotal role in maintaining your well-being.

This cookbook is designed to empower you with a collection of 50 delectable and asthma-friendly recipes that not only tantalize your taste buds but also support your lung health. Each recipe is thoughtfully curated to minimize potential triggers and enhance your overall quality of life.

Living with asthma should never mean sacrificing the joy of savoring delicious meals. Here, you'll discover a diverse range of dishes, from vibrant salads to hearty main courses and delightful snacks, all carefully crafted to align with asthma-friendly guidelines. Our recipes focus on fresh, wholesome ingredients, incorporating foods rich in antioxidants, anti-inflammatory properties, and essential nutrients that support lung function.

Whether you're seeking inspiration for a quick weeknight dinner, planning a family gathering, or simply looking for nutritious and flavorful options, "Breathing Easy" has you covered. We believe that nurturing your body through mindful, asthma-friendly cooking can lead to a happier, healthier life.

As you embark on this culinary adventure, we encourage you to embrace the joy of cooking, share these recipes with loved ones, and savor the flavors that contribute to your well-being. Together, we can make mealtime a celebration of both taste and health, allowing you to breathe easy and savor every moment.

Here's to your culinary journey toward asthma wellness and to "Breathing Easy" with every delightful bite.

# ASTHMA-FRIENDLY RECIPES

**Recipe 1: Grilled Chicken and Veggie Wrap**

**Prep Time:** 20 minutes **Serves:** 2

## Ingredients:

- 2 boneless, skinless chicken breasts

- 1 zucchini, sliced into thin strips

- 1 red bell pepper, sliced

- 1 yellow bell pepper, sliced

- 2 whole wheat tortillas

- 2 tablespoons olive oil

- 1 teaspoon garlic powder

- Salt and pepper to taste

## Directions:

1. Preheat a grill or grill pan to medium-high heat.

2. Season chicken breasts with garlic powder, salt, and pepper.

3. Grill chicken for 6-8 minutes per side or until cooked through.

4. In a separate pan, sauté zucchini and bell peppers in olive oil until tender.

5. Slice grilled chicken into thin strips.

6. Warm tortillas on the grill for about 30 seconds on each side.

7. Lay out each tortilla and fill with sliced chicken and sautéed vegetables.

8. Roll up the tortillas tightly, securing with toothpicks if needed.

9. Slice in half and serve.

**Nutritional Value (per serving):**

- Calories: 350

- Protein: 30g

- Carbohydrates: 20g

- Fiber: 5g

- Fat: 16g

**Recipe 2: Quinoa and Black Bean Salad**

**Prep Time:** 15 minutes **Serves:** 4

**Ingredients:**

- 1 cup quinoa, rinsed and drained

- 2 cups water

- 1 can (15 oz) black beans, drained and rinsed

- 1 cup cherry tomatoes, halved

- 1/2 red onion, finely chopped

- 1/4 cup fresh cilantro, chopped

- Juice of 1 lime

- 2 tablespoons olive oil

- Salt and pepper to taste

**Directions:**

1. In a medium saucepan, bring water to a boil and add quinoa. Reduce heat to low, cover, and simmer for 12-15 minutes or until quinoa is cooked and water is absorbed.

2. Fluff quinoa with a fork and let it cool.

3.  In a large bowl, combine quinoa, black beans, cherry tomatoes, red onion, and cilantro.

4.  In a small bowl, whisk together lime juice, olive oil, salt, and pepper.

5.  Pour the dressing over the salad and toss to combine.

6.  Serve chilled.

**Nutritional Value (per serving):**

- Calories: 270

- Protein: 8g

- Carbohydrates: 45g

- Fiber: 9g

- Fat: 7g

**Recipe 3: Baked Salmon with Lemon-Dill Sauce**

**Prep Time:** 25 minutes **Serves:** 2

**Ingredients:**

- 2 salmon fillets

- 1 lemon, sliced

- 2 tablespoons fresh dill, chopped

- 2 tablespoons olive oil

- 1 clove garlic, minced

- Salt and pepper to taste

**Directions:**

1. Preheat the oven to 375°F (190°C).

2. Place salmon fillets on a baking sheet lined with parchment paper.

3. Drizzle olive oil over the salmon and season with salt, pepper, and minced garlic.

4. Lay lemon slices on top of the salmon.

5. Bake for 15-20 minutes or until the salmon flakes easily with a fork.

6. While the salmon is baking, mix fresh dill with a tablespoon of olive oil.

7. Once the salmon is done, drizzle the dill sauce over it.

8. Serve with steamed vegetables or a side salad.

**Nutritional Value (per serving):**

- Calories: 350

- Protein: 30g

- Carbohydrates: 2g

- Fiber: 1g

- Fat: 25g

**Recipe 4: Spinach and Mushroom Stuffed Chicken Breast**

**Prep Time:** 30 minutes **Serves:** 2

**Ingredients:**

- 2 boneless, skinless chicken breasts

- 2 cups fresh spinach leaves

- 1 cup mushrooms, sliced

- 1/2 cup low-fat cream cheese

- 2 cloves garlic, minced

- 1 tablespoon olive oil

- Salt and pepper to taste

**Directions:**

1. Preheat the oven to 375°F (190°C).

2. In a skillet, heat olive oil over medium heat.

3. Sauté mushrooms and garlic until mushrooms are tender, about 5 minutes.

4. Stir in fresh spinach and cook until wilted. Remove from heat.

5. Make a pocket in each chicken breast by carefully slicing horizontally.

6. Season chicken with salt and pepper.

7. Stuff each chicken breast with the mushroom and spinach mixture, then spread cream cheese over the top.

8. Place stuffed chicken breasts in a baking dish and bake for 20-25 minutes or until chicken is cooked through.

**Nutritional Value (per serving):**

- Calories: 350

- Protein: 30g

- Carbohydrates: 6g

- Fiber: 2g

- Fat: 22g

**Recipe 5: Lentil and Vegetable Soup**

**Prep Time:** 40 minutes **Serves:** 6

**Ingredients:**

- 1 cup green or brown lentils, rinsed

- 6 cups vegetable broth

- 2 carrots, diced

- 2 celery stalks, diced

- 1 onion, chopped

- 2 cloves garlic, minced

- 1 can (15 oz) diced tomatoes

- 1 teaspoon cumin

- 1 teaspoon paprika

- Salt and pepper to taste

- Fresh parsley for garnish

**Directions:**

1. In a large pot, heat olive oil over medium heat.

2. Add onions, carrots, and celery. Sauté for 5-7 minutes until softened.

3. Stir in garlic, cumin, and paprika. Cook for another minute.

4. Add lentils, vegetable broth, and diced tomatoes. Bring to a boil.

5. Reduce heat, cover, and simmer for 25-30 minutes or until lentils are tender.

6. Season with salt and pepper to taste.

7. Garnish with fresh parsley before serving.

**Nutritional Value (per serving):**

- Calories: 200

- Protein: 10g

- Carbohydrates: 36g

- Fiber: 12g

- Fat: 2g

**Recipe 6: Grilled Vegetable and Quinoa Bowl**

**Prep Time:** 25 minutes **Serves:** 4

**Ingredients:**

- 2 cups cooked quinoa

- 2 zucchinis, sliced lengthwise

- 2 bell peppers, quartered

- 1 red onion, cut into rings

- 1 cup cherry tomatoes

- 1/4 cup balsamic vinegar

- 2 tablespoons olive oil

- 1 teaspoon dried oregano

- Salt and pepper to taste

- Fresh basil leaves for garnish

**Directions:**

1. Preheat grill to medium-high heat.

2. In a bowl, whisk together balsamic vinegar, olive oil, dried oregano, salt, and pepper.

3. Brush the marinade onto zucchinis, bell peppers, red onion, and cherry tomatoes.

4. Grill vegetables for 3-5 minutes per side or until they have grill marks and are tender.

5. Arrange cooked quinoa in bowls.

6. Top with grilled vegetables and garnish with fresh basil leaves.

**Nutritional Value (per serving):**

- Calories: 250

- Protein: 6g

- Carbohydrates: 40g

- Fiber: 6g

- Fat: 8g

**Recipe 7: Creamy Tomato Basil Soup**

**Prep Time:** 30 minutes **Serves:** 4

**Ingredients:**

- 1 can (28 oz) crushed tomatoes

- 1 onion, chopped

- 2 cloves garlic, minced

- 1 cup low-sodium vegetable broth

- 1/2 cup unsweetened almond milk

- 1/4 cup fresh basil leaves, chopped

- 2 tablespoons olive oil

- Salt and pepper to taste

**Directions:**

1.  In a large pot, heat olive oil over medium heat.

2.  Add chopped onions and garlic. Sauté for 5-7 minutes until onions are translucent.

3.  Stir in crushed tomatoes, vegetable broth, and almond milk. Bring to a simmer.

4.  Cook for 15-20 minutes, stirring occasionally.

5.  Blend the soup using an immersion blender or a regular blender until smooth.

6.  Return the soup to the pot and stir in chopped basil.

7.  Season with salt and pepper to taste.

8.  Serve hot.

**Nutritional Value (per serving):**

- Calories: 160

- Protein: 4g

- Carbohydrates: 18g

- Fiber: 4g

- Fat: 9g

## Recipe 8: Roasted Butternut Squash and Apple Salad

**Prep Time:** 35 minutes **Serves:** 4

## Ingredients:

- 1 butternut squash, peeled and cubed

- 2 apples, cored and sliced

- 1/4 cup walnuts, chopped

- 4 cups mixed greens

- 2 tablespoons olive oil

- 2 tablespoons balsamic vinegar

- 1 teaspoon honey

- Salt and pepper to taste

## Directions:

1. Preheat the oven to 400°F (200°C).

2. Toss butternut squash cubes with olive oil, salt, and pepper.

3. Spread squash on a baking sheet and roast for 20-25 minutes or until tender.

4. In a small bowl, whisk together balsamic vinegar and honey.

5. In a large salad bowl, combine roasted butternut squash, apple slices, mixed greens, and chopped walnuts.

6. Drizzle the balsamic-honey dressing over the salad and toss gently.

7. Serve immediately.

**Nutritional Value (per serving):**

- Calories: 250

- Protein: 4g

- Carbohydrates: 35g

- Fiber: 7g

- Fat: 12g

**Recipe 9: Sweet Potato and Black Bean Enchiladas**

**Prep Time:** 45 minutes **Serves:** 4

**Ingredients:**

- 2 medium sweet potatoes, peeled and diced

- 1 can (15 oz) black beans, drained and rinsed

- 1 cup corn kernels (fresh or frozen)

- 1 cup diced red bell pepper

- 1 cup diced onion

- 2 cloves garlic, minced

- 1 teaspoon cumin

- 1 teaspoon chili powder

- 8 whole wheat tortillas

- 1 1/2 cups enchilada sauce

- 1 cup shredded cheddar cheese (optional)

- Fresh cilantro for garnish

**Directions:**

1. Preheat the oven to 375°F (190°C).

2. Steam or boil sweet potato cubes until tender, about 10 minutes.

3. In a large skillet, sauté onion, garlic, and red bell pepper until softened.

4. Add cooked sweet potatoes, black beans, corn, cumin, and chili powder to the skillet. Stir to combine.

5. Pour a small amount of enchilada sauce into the bottom of a baking dish.

6. Fill each tortilla with the sweet potato and black bean mixture and roll it up. Place seam side down in the baking dish.

7. Pour remaining enchilada sauce over the top and sprinkle with cheese (if using).

8. Bake for 20-25 minutes or until the enchiladas are heated through and the cheese is bubbly.

9. Garnish with fresh cilantro before serving.

**Nutritional Value (per serving):**

- Calories: 400

- Protein: 12g

- Carbohydrates: 75g

- Fiber: 12g

- Fat: 8g

**Recipe 10: Mediterranean Chickpea Salad**

**Prep Time:** 20 minutes **Serves:** 4

**Ingredients:**

- 2 cans (15 oz each) chickpeas, drained and rinsed

- 1 cucumber, diced

- 1 cup cherry tomatoes, halved

- 1/2 red onion, finely chopped

- 1/4 cup Kalamata olives, pitted and sliced

- 1/4 cup feta cheese, crumbled

- 2 tablespoons olive oil

- 2 tablespoons lemon juice

- 1 teaspoon dried oregano

- Salt and pepper to taste

- Fresh parsley for garnish

## Directions:

1. In a large bowl, combine chickpeas, cucumber, cherry tomatoes, red onion, olives, and feta cheese.

2. In a separate bowl, whisk together olive oil, lemon juice, dried oregano, salt, and pepper.

3. Pour the dressing over the salad and toss to combine.

4. Garnish with fresh parsley before serving.

## Nutritional Value (per serving):

- Calories: 320

- Protein: 14g

- Carbohydrates: 42g

- Fiber: 10g

- Fat: 12g

**Recipe 11: Lemon Garlic Shrimp and Asparagus**

**Prep Time:** 20 minutes **Serves:** 2

**Ingredients:**

- 12 large shrimp, peeled and deveined

- 1 bunch asparagus, trimmed

- 2 cloves garlic, minced

- Zest and juice of 1 lemon

- 2 tablespoons olive oil

- Salt and pepper to taste

- Fresh parsley for garnish

**Directions:**

1. Preheat the oven to 400°F (200°C).

2. In a bowl, mix together olive oil, minced garlic, lemon zest, lemon juice, salt, and pepper.

3.  Toss asparagus with half of the lemon-garlic mixture and spread on a baking sheet.

4.  Roast asparagus for 10-12 minutes until tender.

5.  In a skillet, heat the remaining lemon-garlic mixture over medium heat.

6.  Add shrimp and cook for 2-3 minutes per side or until pink and cooked through.

7.  Serve shrimp over roasted asparagus and garnish with fresh parsley.

**Nutritional Value (per serving):**

- Calories: 250

- Protein: 24g

- Carbohydrates: 10g

- Fiber: 4g

- Fat: 14g

**Recipe 12: Creamy Avocado and Spinach Pasta**

**Prep Time:** 20 minutes **Serves:** 4

**Ingredients:**

- 8 oz whole wheat pasta

- 2 ripe avocados

- 2 cups fresh spinach

- 1/4 cup fresh basil leaves

- 2 cloves garlic, minced

- Juice of 1 lemon

- 1/4 cup grated Parmesan cheese

- Salt and pepper to taste

**Directions:**

1. Cook pasta according to package instructions.

2. In a blender or food processor, combine avocados, spinach, basil, garlic, lemon juice, Parmesan cheese, salt, and pepper.

3. Blend until smooth and creamy.

4. Toss the cooked pasta with the avocado sauce until well coated.

5. Serve immediately.

**Nutritional Value (per serving):**

- Calories: 350

- Protein: 10g

- Carbohydrates: 45g

- Fiber: 8g

- Fat: 15g

**Recipe 13: Turkey and Vegetable Stir-Fry**

Prep Time: 25 minutes Serves: 4

**Ingredients:**

- 1 lb ground turkey

- 2 cups broccoli florets

- 1 bell pepper, sliced

- 1 carrot, thinly sliced

- 1/2 cup snap peas, trimmed

- 2 cloves garlic, minced

- 2 tablespoons low-sodium soy sauce

- 1 tablespoon honey

- 1 teaspoon ginger, minced

- 2 tablespoons olive oil

- Salt and pepper to taste

**Directions:**

1. In a small bowl, whisk together soy sauce, honey, and ginger.

2. In a large skillet or wok, heat olive oil over high heat.

3. Add ground turkey and garlic. Stir-fry until turkey is cooked through and browned.

4. Remove turkey from the skillet and set aside.

5. In the same skillet, add more oil if needed and stir-fry broccoli, bell pepper, carrot, and snap peas until they are tender-crisp.

6. Return the cooked turkey to the skillet and pour the sauce over the mixture.

7. Stir-fry for an additional 2-3 minutes until everything is heated through.

8. Season with salt and pepper to taste.

9. Serve hot.

**Nutritional Value (per serving):**

- Calories: 300

- Protein: 25g

- Carbohydrates: 15g

- Fiber: 4g

- Fat: 15g

**Recipe 14: Zucchini Noodles with Pesto and Cherry Tomatoes**

**Prep Time:** 20 minutes **Serves:** 2

**Ingredients:**

- 2 large zucchinis, spiralized into noodles

- 1 cup cherry tomatoes, halved

- 1/4 cup pesto sauce (store-bought or homemade)

- 1/4 cup pine nuts, toasted

- Grated Parmesan cheese for garnish

- Salt and pepper to taste

**Directions:**

1. In a large skillet, heat olive oil over medium heat.

2. Add cherry tomatoes and cook for 2-3 minutes until they start to soften.

3. Stir in zucchini noodles and cook for another 2-3 minutes until they are heated through but still crisp.

4.  Remove from heat and toss with pesto sauce.

5.  Season with salt and pepper to taste.

6.  Serve topped with toasted pine nuts and grated Parmesan cheese.

**Nutritional Value (per serving):**

- Calories: 320

- Protein: 8g

- Carbohydrates: 14g

- Fiber: 4g

- Fat: 26g

**Recipe 15: Roasted Red Pepper Hummus**

**Prep Time:** 15 minutes **Serves:** 6

**Ingredients:**

- 1 can (15 oz) chickpeas, drained and rinsed

- 1/2 cup roasted red peppers, drained

- 2 cloves garlic, minced

- 2 tablespoons tahini

- Juice of 1 lemon

- 2 tablespoons olive oil

- 1/2 teaspoon cumin

- Salt and pepper to taste

- Fresh parsley for garnish

**Directions:**

1. In a food processor, combine chickpeas, roasted red peppers, garlic, tahini, lemon juice, olive oil, cumin, salt, and pepper.

2. Blend until smooth and creamy, scraping down the sides as needed.

3. Transfer to a serving bowl and garnish with fresh parsley.

4. Serve with whole wheat pita bread or vegetable sticks.

**Nutritional Value (per serving):**

- Calories: 150

- Protein: 5g

- Carbohydrates: 15g

- Fiber: 4g

- Fat: 8g

**Recipe 16: Teriyaki Tofu and Vegetable Skewers**

**Prep Time:** 30 minutes **Serves:** 4

**Ingredients:**

- 1 block extra-firm tofu, cubed

- 1 bell pepper, cut into chunks

- 1 zucchini, sliced into rounds

- 1 red onion, cut into wedges

- 1 cup pineapple chunks (fresh or canned)

- 1/4 cup low-sodium teriyaki sauce

- 2 tablespoons olive oil

- Salt and pepper to taste

- Wooden skewers, soaked in water

**Directions:**

1. In a bowl, combine teriyaki sauce, olive oil, salt, and pepper.

2. Thread tofu, bell pepper, zucchini, red onion, and pineapple onto the soaked wooden skewers.

3. Brush skewers with the teriyaki marinade.

4. Preheat grill to medium-high heat.

5. Grill skewers for 5-7 minutes per side or until tofu is heated through and vegetables are tender.

6. Serve hot with additional teriyaki sauce for dipping.

**Nutritional Value (per serving):**

- Calories: 250

- Protein: 12g

- Carbohydrates: 20g

- Fiber: 4g

- Fat: 14g

**Recipe 17: Eggplant and Tomato Stew**

**Prep Time:** 35 minutes **Serves:** 4

**Ingredients:**

- 1 large eggplant, diced

- 2 cups diced tomatoes (canned or fresh)

- 1 onion, chopped

- 2 cloves garlic, minced

- 1 red bell pepper, diced

- 1/2 cup low-sodium vegetable broth

- 1 teaspoon dried basil

- 1 teaspoon dried oregano

- 2 tablespoons olive oil

- Salt and pepper to taste

- Fresh basil leaves for garnish

## Directions:

1. In a large pot, heat olive oil over medium heat.

2. Add chopped onions and garlic. Sauté for 5-7 minutes until onions are translucent.

3. Stir in diced eggplant and red bell pepper. Cook for another 5 minutes.

4. Add diced tomatoes, vegetable broth, dried basil, dried oregano, salt, and pepper.

5. Reduce heat, cover, and simmer for 20-25 minutes or until eggplant is tender.

6. Garnish with fresh basil leaves before serving.

## Nutritional Value (per serving):

- Calories: 180

- Protein: 3g

- Carbohydrates: 28g

- Fiber: 8g

- Fat: 7g

**Recipe 18: Sweet and Spicy Glazed Salmon**

**Prep Time:** 25 minutes **Serves:** 2

**Ingredients:**

- 2 salmon fillets

- 1/4 cup honey

- 2 tablespoons low-sodium soy sauce

- 1 tablespoon Sriracha sauce

- 1 teaspoon minced ginger

- 2 cloves garlic, minced

- 1 tablespoon olive oil

- Salt and pepper to taste

- Sesame seeds for garnish

- Sliced green onions for garnish

## Directions:

1. In a small bowl, whisk together honey, soy sauce, Sriracha sauce, minced ginger, and minced garlic.

2. Season salmon fillets with salt and pepper.

3. In a skillet, heat olive oil over medium-high heat.

4. Add salmon fillets and cook for 3-4 minutes per side.

5. Pour the honey-soy glaze over the salmon and cook for an additional 1-2 minutes until the glaze thickens.

6. Garnish with sesame seeds and sliced green onions before serving.

## Nutritional Value (per serving):

- Calories: 350

- Protein: 30g

- Carbohydrates: 22g

- Fiber: 1g

- Fat: 16g

## Recipe 19: Vegan Lentil and Mushroom Shepherd's Pie

**Prep Time:** 45 minutes **Serves:** 6

## Ingredients:

- 1 cup green or brown lentils, rinsed

- 3 cups vegetable broth

- 1 onion, chopped

- 2 cloves garlic, minced

- 2 carrots, diced

- 2 celery stalks, diced

- 8 oz mushrooms, chopped

- 2 tablespoons tomato paste

- 1 teaspoon dried thyme

- 1 teaspoon dried rosemary

- Salt and pepper to taste

- 4 cups mashed sweet potatoes (made with a touch of olive oil and almond milk)

- Fresh parsley for garnish

**Directions:**

1. In a large pot, combine lentils and vegetable broth. Bring to a boil, then reduce heat and simmer for 20-25 minutes until lentils are tender.

2. In a skillet, heat olive oil over medium heat.

3. Add chopped onions, garlic, carrots, and celery. Sauté for 5-7 minutes until vegetables are softened.

4. Stir in mushrooms and cook for another 5 minutes.

5. Add tomato paste, dried thyme, dried rosemary, salt, and pepper to the skillet. Cook for 2 minutes.

6. Preheat the oven to 375°F (190°C).

7. Combine the cooked lentils and the mushroom mixture in a baking dish.

8. Spread the mashed sweet potatoes over the top.

9. Bake for 20-25 minutes until the top is lightly browned.

10. Garnish with fresh parsley before serving.

**Nutritional Value (per serving):**

- Calories: 300

- Protein: 12g

- Carbohydrates: 55g

- Fiber: 12g

- Fat: 5g

**Recipe 20: Caprese Stuffed Portobello Mushrooms**

**Prep Time:** 30 minutes **Serves:** 4

**Ingredients:**

- 4 large Portobello mushrooms

- 1 cup cherry tomatoes, halved

- 1/2 cup fresh mozzarella cheese, diced

- 1/4 cup fresh basil leaves, chopped

- 2 cloves garlic, minced

- 2 tablespoons balsamic vinegar

- 2 tablespoons olive oil

- Salt and pepper to taste

**Directions:**

1. Preheat the oven to 375°F (190°C).

2. Remove the stems from the Portobello mushrooms and clean the caps.

3. In a bowl, combine cherry tomatoes, fresh mozzarella, chopped basil, minced garlic, balsamic vinegar, olive oil, salt, and pepper.

4. Spoon the tomato and mozzarella mixture into the mushroom caps.

5. Place stuffed mushrooms on a baking sheet and bake for 20-25 minutes until mushrooms are tender and cheese is melted.

6. Serve hot.

**Nutritional Value (per serving):**

- Calories: 200

- Protein: 8g

- Carbohydrates: 10g

- Fiber: 2g

- Fat: 15g

**Recipe 21: Chickpea and Vegetable Curry**
**Prep Time:** 35 minutes **Serves:** 4

**Ingredients:**

- 2 cans (15 oz each) chickpeas, drained and rinsed

- 1 onion, chopped

- 2 cloves garlic, minced

- 1 bell pepper, diced

- 1 zucchini, diced

- 1 can (14 oz) diced tomatoes

- 1 can (14 oz) coconut milk

- 2 tablespoons olive oil

- 2 tablespoons curry powder

- 1 teaspoon ground cumin

- Salt and pepper to taste

- Fresh cilantro for garnish

## Directions:

1. In a large skillet, heat olive oil over medium heat.

2. Add chopped onions and garlic. Sauté for 5-7 minutes until onions are translucent.

3. Stir in curry powder and ground cumin. Cook for 2 minutes.

4. Add diced bell pepper and zucchini. Cook for another 5 minutes.

5. Pour in diced tomatoes (with juice), coconut milk, chickpeas, salt, and pepper. Stir to combine.

6. Simmer for 15-20 minutes until the vegetables are tender and the curry has thickened.

7. Garnish with fresh cilantro before serving.

## Nutritional Value (per serving):

- Calories: 350

- Protein: 10g

- Carbohydrates: 30g

- Fiber: 9g

- Fat: 22g

## Recipe 22: Almond-Crusted Baked Chicken Tenders

**Prep Time:** 30 minutes **Serves:** 4

## Ingredients:

- 1 lb chicken tenders

- 1 cup almond meal

- 1/2 teaspoon paprika

- 1/2 teaspoon garlic powder

- 1/4 teaspoon cayenne pepper

- 1/4 cup almond milk

- 1 egg

- Salt and pepper to taste

- Cooking spray

## Directions:

1. Preheat the oven to 400°F (200°C).

2. In a shallow bowl, combine almond meal, paprika, garlic powder, cayenne pepper, salt, and pepper.

3. In another shallow bowl, whisk together almond milk and egg.

4. Dip each chicken tender into the almond milk mixture, then coat with almond meal mixture, pressing firmly to adhere.

5. Place the coated chicken tenders on a baking sheet lined with parchment paper.

6. Spray the chicken tenders with cooking spray.

7. Bake for 20-25 minutes until chicken is cooked through and coating is crispy.

8. Serve with your favorite dipping sauce.

**Nutritional Value (per serving):**

- Calories: 250

- Protein: 30g

- Carbohydrates: 6g

- Fiber: 3g

- Fat: 12g

**Recipe 23: Roasted Beet and Goat Cheese Salad**

**Prep Time:** 40 minutes **Serves:** 4

**Ingredients:**

- 4 medium beets, peeled and cubed

- 4 cups mixed salad greens

- 4 oz goat cheese, crumbled

- 1/4 cup walnuts, chopped and toasted

- 2 tablespoons balsamic vinegar

- 2 tablespoons olive oil

- 1 teaspoon honey

- Salt and pepper to taste

**Directions:**

1. Preheat the oven to 400°F (200°C).

2. Toss beet cubes with olive oil, salt, and pepper.

3. Spread beets on a baking sheet and roast for 25-30 minutes until tender.

4. In a small bowl, whisk together balsamic vinegar, honey, salt, and pepper.

5. Arrange salad greens on serving plates.

6. Top with roasted beets, crumbled goat cheese, and toasted walnuts.

7. Drizzle the balsamic dressing over the salad.

8. Serve immediately.

**Nutritional Value (per serving):**

- Calories: 250

- Protein: 8g

- Carbohydrates: 20g

- Fiber: 5g

- Fat: 15g

## Recipe 24: Spinach and Feta Stuffed Mushrooms

**Prep Time:** 25 minutes **Serves:** 4

**Ingredients:**

- 12 large button mushrooms, stems removed
- 2 cups fresh spinach, chopped
- 1/2 cup feta cheese, crumbled
- 2 cloves garlic, minced
- 2 tablespoons olive oil
- Salt and pepper to taste

**Directions:**

1. Preheat the oven to 375°F (190°C).
2. In a skillet, heat olive oil over medium heat.
3. Add minced garlic and chopped spinach. Sauté for 2-3 minutes until spinach is wilted.
4. Remove from heat and stir in crumbled feta cheese.
5. Stuff each mushroom cap with the spinach and feta mixture.
6. Place stuffed mushrooms on a baking sheet.

7. Bake for 15-20 minutes until mushrooms are tender and filling is heated through.

8. Serve hot.

## Nutritional Value (per serving):

- Calories: 120

- Protein: 4g

- Carbohydrates: 4g

- Fiber: 1g

- Fat: 10g

## Recipe 25: Blueberry and Almond Overnight Oats

**Prep Time:** 10 minutes (plus overnight refrigeration) **Serves:** 2

## Ingredients:

- 1 cup rolled oats

- 1 cup unsweetened almond milk

- 1/2 cup fresh blueberries

- 1/4 cup sliced almonds

- 2 tablespoons honey

- 1/2 teaspoon vanilla extract

- Pinch of salt

## Directions:

1. In a mixing bowl, combine rolled oats, almond milk, honey, vanilla extract, and a pinch of salt.

2. Divide the mixture between two jars or containers.

3. Top each jar with fresh blueberries and sliced almonds.

4. Seal the jars and refrigerate overnight.

5. In the morning, give the oats a good stir and enjoy a delicious, no-cook breakfast!

## Nutritional Value (per serving):

- Calories: 300

- Protein: 7g

- Carbohydrates: 50g

- Fiber: 7g

- Fat: 10g

### Recipe 26: Quinoa and Roasted Vegetable Bowl

**Prep Time:** 40 minutes **Serves:** 4

**Ingredients:**

- 1 cup quinoa, rinsed and drained

- 2 cups mixed vegetables (e.g., bell peppers, broccoli, carrots), chopped

- 2 tablespoons olive oil

- 1 teaspoon dried thyme

- 1/2 teaspoon smoked paprika

- Salt and pepper to taste

- 1/4 cup fresh parsley, chopped

- 1/4 cup balsamic vinaigrette dressing (store-bought or homemade)

**Directions:**

1. Preheat the oven to 400°F (200°C).

2. Toss the mixed vegetables with olive oil, dried thyme, smoked paprika, salt, and pepper.

3. Spread the vegetables on a baking sheet and roast for 20-25 minutes or until they are tender and slightly caramelized.

4. While the vegetables roast, cook quinoa according to package instructions.

5. In a large bowl, combine cooked quinoa and roasted vegetables.

6. Drizzle with balsamic vinaigrette dressing and toss to coat.

7. Garnish with fresh parsley before serving.

**Nutritional Value (per serving):**

- Calories: 280

- Protein: 6g

- Carbohydrates: 42g

- Fiber: 6g

- Fat: 10g

## Recipe 27: Lemon Herb Baked Salmon

**Prep Time:** 25 minutes **Serves:** 2

**Ingredients:**

- 2 salmon fillets

- Zest and juice of 1 lemon

- 2 cloves garlic, minced

- 1 tablespoon olive oil

- 1 teaspoon dried dill

- Salt and pepper to taste

- Fresh dill for garnish

**Directions:**

1. Preheat the oven to 375°F (190°C).

2. In a small bowl, whisk together lemon zest, lemon juice, minced garlic, olive oil, dried dill, salt, and pepper.

3. Place salmon fillets on a baking sheet lined with parchment paper.

4. Brush the lemon herb mixture over the salmon.

5. Bake for 15-20 minutes or until the salmon flakes easily with a fork.

6. Garnish with fresh dill before serving.

## Nutritional Value (per serving):

- Calories: 300

- Protein: 30g

- Carbohydrates: 2g

- Fiber: 0g

- Fat: 20g

**Recipe 28: Black Bean and Corn Salsa**

**Prep Time:** 15 minutes **Serves:** 4

## Ingredients:

- 1 can (15 oz) black beans, drained and rinsed

- 1 cup corn kernels (fresh or frozen)

- 1/2 red onion, finely chopped

- 1 bell pepper, diced

- 1 jalapeño pepper, seeded and minced (optional for heat)

- Juice of 2 limes

- 2 tablespoons fresh cilantro, chopped

- Salt and pepper to taste

- Tortilla chips or whole-grain crackers for serving

**Directions:**

1. In a large bowl, combine black beans, corn, chopped red onion, diced bell pepper, and minced jalapeño pepper (if using).

2. Squeeze the juice of two limes over the mixture.

3. Add chopped cilantro, salt, and pepper.

4. Mix well and refrigerate for at least 30 minutes before serving.

5. Serve with tortilla chips or whole-grain crackers.

**Nutritional Value (per serving):**

- Calories: 180

- Protein: 8g

- Carbohydrates: 36g

- Fiber: 10g

- Fat: 1g

**Recipe 29: Cucumber and Dill Greek Yogurt Dip**

**Prep Time:** 10 minutes **Serves:** 4

**Ingredients:**

- 1 cucumber, finely grated

- 1 cup Greek yogurt

- 2 cloves garlic, minced

- 1 tablespoon fresh dill, chopped

- Juice of 1 lemon

- Salt and pepper to taste

- Vegetable sticks (carrots, celery, cucumbers) for dipping

**Directions:**

1. Place the grated cucumber in a clean kitchen towel and squeeze out excess moisture.

2. In a bowl, combine grated cucumber, Greek yogurt, minced garlic, chopped dill, lemon juice, salt, and pepper.

3.  Mix well and refrigerate for at least 30 minutes before serving.

4.  Serve with vegetable sticks for dipping.

**Nutritional Value (per serving):**

- Calories: 60

- Protein: 5g

- Carbohydrates: 7g

- Fiber: 1g

- Fat: 1g

**Recipe 30: Baked Sweet Potato Fries**

**Prep Time:** 30 minutes **Serves:** 4

**Ingredients:**

- 2 large sweet potatoes, cut into fries

- 2 tablespoons olive oil

- 1 teaspoon paprika

- 1/2 teaspoon garlic powder

- 1/2 teaspoon onion powder

- Salt and pepper to taste

- Fresh parsley for garnish

**Directions:**

1. Preheat the oven to 425°F (220°C).

2. In a large bowl, toss sweet potato fries with olive oil, paprika, garlic powder, onion powder, salt, and pepper.

3. Spread the fries in a single layer on a baking sheet.

4. Bake for 25-30 minutes, flipping once, until fries are crispy and golden.

5. Garnish with fresh parsley before serving.

**Nutritional Value (per serving):**

- Calories: 150

- Protein: 2g

- Carbohydrates: 23g

- Fiber: 4g

- Fat: 6g

**Recipe 31: Ginger Turmeric Tea**

**Prep Time:** 10 minutes **Serves:** 2

**Ingredients:**

- 2 cups water

- 1-inch piece of fresh ginger, sliced

- 1/2 teaspoon ground turmeric

- Honey or maple syrup to taste (optional)

**Directions:**

1. In a small pot, bring 2 cups of water to a boil.

2. Add sliced ginger and ground turmeric to the boiling water.

3. Reduce heat and simmer for 5-7 minutes.

4. Strain the tea into cups.

5. Sweeten with honey or maple syrup if desired.

**Nutritional Value (per serving):**

- Calories: 0

- Protein: 0g

- Carbohydrates: 0g

- Fiber: 0g

- Fat: 0g

**Recipe 32: Mediterranean Stuffed Bell Peppers**

**Prep Time:** 50 minutes **Serves:** 4

**Ingredients:**

- 4 bell peppers, any color

- 1 cup cooked quinoa

- 1 can (15 oz) chickpeas, drained and rinsed

- 1/2 cup diced cucumber

- 1/2 cup diced tomatoes

- 1/4 cup Kalamata olives, pitted and sliced

- 1/4 cup crumbled feta cheese

- 2 tablespoons olive oil

- Juice of 1 lemon

- 1 teaspoon dried oregano

- Salt and pepper to taste

- Fresh parsley for garnish

## Directions:

1.  Preheat the oven to 375°F (190°C).

2.  Cut the tops off the bell peppers and remove seeds and membranes.

3.  In a large bowl, combine cooked quinoa, chickpeas, diced cucumber, diced tomatoes, sliced Kalamata olives, crumbled feta cheese, olive oil, lemon juice, dried oregano, salt, and pepper.

4.  Stuff each bell pepper with the quinoa mixture.

5.  Place stuffed peppers in a baking dish.

6.  Cover with aluminum foil and bake for 30-35 minutes until peppers are tender.

7.  Garnish with fresh parsley before serving.

## Nutritional Value (per serving):

- Calories: 300

- Protein: 10g

- Carbohydrates: 42g

- Fiber: 10g

- Fat: 12g

**Recipe 33: Coconut Banana Smoothie**

**Prep Time:** 5 minutes **Serves:** 2

**Ingredients:**

- 2 ripe bananas

- 1 cup coconut milk

- 1/2 cup Greek yogurt

- 1 tablespoon honey

- 1/2 teaspoon vanilla extract

- 1/4 teaspoon ground cinnamon

- Ice cubes (optional)

- Unsweetened shredded coconut for garnish (optional)

**Directions:**

1. Place ripe bananas, coconut milk, Greek yogurt, honey, vanilla extract, and ground cinnamon in a blender.

2. Add ice cubes if you prefer a colder smoothie.

3. Blend until smooth and creamy.

4. Pour into glasses and garnish with unsweetened shredded coconut if desired.

**Nutritional Value (per serving):**

- Calories: 200

- Protein: 4g

- Carbohydrates: 35g

- Fiber: 3g

- Fat: 8g

**Recipe 34: Tomato Basil Quinoa Salad**

**Prep Time:** 30 minutes **Serves:** 4

**Ingredients:**

- 1 cup quinoa, rinsed and drained

- 2 cups cherry tomatoes, halved

- 1/2 cup fresh basil leaves, chopped

- 1/4 cup red onion, finely chopped

- 2 cloves garlic, minced

- 2 tablespoons olive oil

- Juice of 1 lemon

- Salt and pepper to taste

## Directions:

1. Cook quinoa according to package instructions.

2. In a large bowl, combine cooked quinoa, cherry tomatoes, chopped basil, chopped red onion, minced garlic, olive oil, lemon juice, salt, and pepper.

3. Toss to combine all ingredients.

4. Serve chilled.

## Nutritional Value (per serving):

- Calories: 250

- Protein: 6g

- Carbohydrates: 38g

- Fiber: 5g

- Fat: 8g

### Recipe 35: Baked Cod with Lemon and Herbs

**Prep Time:** 30 minutes **Serves:** 2

## Ingredients:

- 2 cod fillets

- Zest and juice of 1 lemon

- 2 cloves garlic, minced

- 1 tablespoon fresh parsley, chopped

- 1 tablespoon fresh dill, chopped

- 1 tablespoon olive oil

- Salt and pepper to taste

- Lemon wedges for garnish

## Directions:

1. Preheat the oven to 375°F (190°C).

2. In a small bowl, combine lemon zest, lemon juice, minced garlic, chopped parsley, chopped dill, olive oil, salt, and pepper.

3. Place cod fillets on a baking sheet lined with parchment paper.

4. Drizzle the lemon and herb mixture over the cod.

5. Bake for 15-20 minutes or until the cod flakes easily with a fork.

6. Garnish with lemon wedges before serving.

## Nutritional Value (per serving):

- Calories: 180

- Protein: 25g

- Carbohydrates: 3g

- Fiber: 0g

- Fat: 7g

**Recipe 36: Mango and Spinach Salad with Citrus Dressing**

**Prep Time:** 20 minutes **Serves:** 4

**Ingredients:**

- 6 cups baby spinach leaves

- 2 ripe mangoes, peeled, pitted, and sliced

- 1/4 cup red onion, thinly sliced

- 1/4 cup sliced almonds, toasted

- 1/4 cup fresh cilantro, chopped

- Juice of 1 orange

- Juice of 1 lime

- 2 tablespoons olive oil

- 1 tablespoon honey

- Salt and pepper to taste

**Directions:**

1. In a large bowl, combine baby spinach, sliced mangoes, thinly sliced red onion, toasted sliced almonds, and chopped cilantro.

2. In a small bowl, whisk together orange juice, lime juice, olive oil, honey, salt, and pepper.

3. Drizzle the citrus dressing over the salad.

4. Toss to coat all ingredients.

5. Serve immediately.

**Nutritional Value (per serving):**

- Calories: 200

- Protein: 3g

- Carbohydrates: 27g

- Fiber: 5g

- Fat: 10g

**Recipe 37: Lemon Herb Quinoa Salad**

**Prep Time:** 25 minutes **Serves:** 4

**Ingredients:**

- 1 cup quinoa, rinsed and drained

- Zest and juice of 1 lemon

- 2 tablespoons fresh parsley, chopped

- 2 tablespoons fresh mint, chopped

- 1/4 cup cherry tomatoes, halved

- 1/4 cup cucumber, diced

- 2 tablespoons olive oil

- Salt and pepper to taste

## Directions:

1. Cook quinoa according to package instructions.

2. In a large bowl, combine cooked quinoa, lemon zest, lemon juice, chopped parsley, chopped mint, cherry tomatoes, diced cucumber, olive oil, salt, and pepper.

3. Toss to combine all ingredients.

4. Serve chilled.

## Nutritional Value (per serving):

- Calories: 200

- Protein: 5g

- Carbohydrates: 28g

- Fiber: 3g

- Fat: 8g

**Recipe 38: Roasted Brussels Sprouts with Balsamic Glaze**

**Prep Time:** 30 minutes **Serves:** 4

## Ingredients:

- 1 lb Brussels sprouts, trimmed and halved

- 2 tablespoons olive oil

- Salt and pepper to taste

- 2 tablespoons balsamic vinegar

- 1 tablespoon honey

- 1/4 cup chopped pecans, toasted (optional)

## Directions:

1. Preheat the oven to 400°F (200°C).

2. Toss Brussels sprouts with olive oil, salt, and pepper.

3. Spread the Brussels sprouts on a baking sheet and roast for 20-25 minutes until they are tender and slightly caramelized.

4. In a small saucepan, heat balsamic vinegar and honey over low heat. Simmer for 2-3 minutes until it thickens into a glaze.

5. Drizzle the balsamic glaze over the roasted Brussels sprouts.

6. If desired, sprinkle with toasted chopped pecans before serving.

## Nutritional Value (per serving):

- Calories: 120

- Protein: 3g

- Carbohydrates: 16g

- Fiber: 4g

- Fat: 6g

### Recipe 39: Vegan Lentil Soup

**Prep Time:** 40 minutes **Serves:** 6

### Ingredients:

- 1 cup green or brown lentils, rinsed

- 8 cups vegetable broth

- 1 onion, chopped

- 2 carrots, diced

- 2 celery stalks, diced

- 2 cloves garlic, minced

- 1 can (14 oz) diced tomatoes

- 1 teaspoon ground cumin

- 1 teaspoon smoked paprika

- Salt and pepper to taste

- Fresh parsley for garnish

**Directions:**

1. In a large pot, combine lentils and vegetable broth. Bring to a boil, then reduce heat and simmer for 20-25 minutes until lentils are tender.

2. In a separate large pot, heat olive oil over medium heat.

3. Add chopped onions, diced carrots, diced celery, and minced garlic. Sauté for 5-7 minutes until vegetables are softened.

4. Stir in diced tomatoes, ground cumin, smoked paprika, salt, and pepper. Cook for 2 minutes.

5. Add the cooked lentils and vegetable broth to the pot with the sautéed vegetables.

6. Simmer for an additional 10-15 minutes to meld the flavors.

7. Garnish with fresh parsley before serving.

**Nutritional Value (per serving):**

- Calories: 250

- Protein: 12g

- Carbohydrates: 42g

- Fiber: 12g

- Fat: 2g

**Recipe 40: Grilled Shrimp and Pineapple Skewers**

**Prep Time:** 30 minutes **Serves:** 4

**Ingredients:**

- 1 lb large shrimp, peeled and deveined

- 2 cups pineapple chunks

- 2 tablespoons olive oil

- 2 cloves garlic, minced

- 1 teaspoon paprika

- 1/2 teaspoon chili powder

- Salt and pepper to taste

- Fresh cilantro for garnish

## Directions:

1. Preheat a grill to medium-high heat.

2. In a bowl, combine olive oil, minced garlic, paprika, chili powder, salt, and pepper.

3. Thread shrimp and pineapple alternately onto skewers.

4. Brush the skewers with the olive oil and spice mixture.

5. Grill for 2-3 minutes per side until the shrimp are pink and opaque.

6. Garnish with fresh cilantro before serving.

## Nutritional Value (per serving):

- Calories: 220

- Protein: 22g

- Carbohydrates: 16g

- Fiber: 2g

- Fat: 8g

**Recipe 41: Turkey and Vegetable Stir-Fry**

**Prep Time:** 30 minutes **Serves:** 4

**Ingredients:**

- 1 lb lean ground turkey

- 2 cups broccoli florets

- 1 red bell pepper, sliced

- 1 yellow bell pepper, sliced

- 1 zucchini, sliced

- 2 cloves garlic, minced

- 2 tablespoons low-sodium soy sauce

- 1 tablespoon hoisin sauce

- 1 teaspoon fresh ginger, minced

- 1 teaspoon sesame oil

- Salt and pepper to taste

- Cooked brown rice for serving

## Directions:

1. In a skillet, cook lean ground turkey over medium-high heat until no longer pink. Break it up into crumbles as it cooks. Remove from the skillet and set aside.

2. In the same skillet, add a bit of olive oil if needed. Add minced garlic and cook for 30 seconds.

3. Add broccoli florets, sliced red bell pepper, sliced yellow bell pepper, and sliced zucchini to the skillet. Stir-fry for 5-7 minutes until the vegetables are tender-crisp.

4. In a small bowl, whisk together low-sodium soy sauce, hoisin sauce, minced ginger, sesame oil, salt, and pepper.

5. Return the cooked turkey to the skillet and pour the sauce over the turkey and vegetables.

6. Stir-fry for an additional 2-3 minutes to heat everything through.

7. Serve over cooked brown rice.

## Nutritional Value (per serving):

- Calories: 250

- Protein: 25g

- Carbohydrates: 18g

- Fiber: 4g

- Fat: 8g

**Recipe 42: Berry and Spinach Smoothie Bowl**

**Prep Time:** 10 minutes **Serves:** 2

**Ingredients:**

- 2 cups fresh spinach leaves

- 1 cup mixed berries (strawberries, blueberries, raspberries)

- 1 ripe banana

- 1/2 cup Greek yogurt

- 1/4 cup unsweetened almond milk

- 2 tablespoons honey

- 1/4 cup granola

- Fresh berries and sliced banana for topping

**Directions:**

1. Place fresh spinach, mixed berries, ripe banana, Greek yogurt, almond milk, and honey in a blender.

2. Blend until smooth and creamy.

3. Divide the smoothie mixture between two bowls.

4. Top with granola, fresh berries, and sliced banana.

5. Serve immediately.

## Nutritional Value (per serving):

- Calories: 250

- Protein: 8g

- Carbohydrates: 50g

- Fiber: 7g

- Fat: 3g

## Recipe 43: Turkey and Black Bean Chili

**Prep Time:** 40 minutes **Serves:** 6

## Ingredients:

- 1 lb ground turkey

- 1 onion, chopped

- 2 cloves garlic, minced

- 1 bell pepper, diced

- 1 can (15 oz) black beans, drained and rinsed

- 1 can (14 oz) diced tomatoes

- 1 cup corn kernels (fresh or frozen)

- 2 tablespoons chili powder

- 1 teaspoon ground cumin

- Salt and pepper to taste

- Fresh cilantro for garnish

- Greek yogurt for topping (optional)

**Directions:**

1. In a large pot, cook ground turkey over medium-high heat until no longer pink. Break it up into crumbles as it cooks. Remove from the pot and set aside.

2. In the same pot, add a bit of olive oil if needed. Add chopped onion, minced garlic, and diced bell pepper. Sauté for 5-7 minutes until vegetables are softened.

3. Return the cooked turkey to the pot.

4. Add drained and rinsed black beans, diced tomatoes (with juice), corn kernels, chili powder, ground cumin, salt, and pepper.

5. Simmer for 20-25 minutes until flavors meld and chili thickens.

6. Garnish with fresh cilantro and a dollop of Greek yogurt if desired.

**Nutritional Value (per serving):**

- Calories: 300

- Protein: 20g

- Carbohydrates: 35g

- Fiber: 8g

- Fat: 10g

**Recipe 44: Caprese Salad with Balsamic Reduction**

**Prep Time:** 15 minutes **Serves:** 4

**Ingredients:**

- 4 large tomatoes, sliced

- 1 cup fresh mozzarella cheese, sliced

- 1/4 cup fresh basil leaves

- 2 tablespoons balsamic reduction (store-bought or homemade)

- 2 tablespoons extra-virgin olive oil

- Salt and pepper to taste

## Directions:

1. Arrange tomato slices, fresh mozzarella slices, and fresh basil leaves on a serving platter.

2. Drizzle with balsamic reduction and extra-virgin olive oil.

3. Season with salt and pepper.

4. Serve immediately.

## Nutritional Value (per serving):

- Calories: 200

- Protein: 10g

- Carbohydrates: 8g

- Fiber: 2g

- Fat: 15g

**Recipe 45: Spaghetti Squash with Pesto**

**Prep Time:** 45 minutes **Serves:** 4

## Ingredients:

- 1 large spaghetti squash
- 1 cup cherry tomatoes, halved
- 1/2 cup pesto sauce (store-bought or homemade)
- 1/4 cup grated Parmesan cheese
- Fresh basil leaves for garnish
- Salt and pepper to taste

## Directions:

1. Preheat the oven to 375°F (190°C).

2. Cut the spaghetti squash in half lengthwise and remove the seeds.

3. Place the squash halves, cut side down, on a baking sheet lined with parchment paper.

4. Bake for 30-35 minutes until the squash is tender and easily shreds into "spaghetti" with a fork.

5. Use a fork to shred the cooked spaghetti squash into a large bowl.

6.  Toss with halved cherry tomatoes and pesto sauce.

7.  Season with salt and pepper.

8.  Sprinkle with grated Parmesan cheese and garnish with fresh basil leaves before serving.

**Nutritional Value (per serving):**

- Calories: 250

- Protein: 5g

- Carbohydrates: 20g

- Fiber: 5g

- Fat: 18g

**Recipe 46: Greek Chicken Souvlaki**

**Prep Time:** 30 minutes **Serves:** 4

**Ingredients:**

- 1 lb boneless, skinless chicken breasts, cut into cubes

- 1/4 cup Greek yogurt

- 2 cloves garlic, minced

- Juice of 1 lemon

- 1 teaspoon dried oregano

- Salt and pepper to taste

- 4 pita bread rounds

- Tzatziki sauce for serving

- Sliced cucumber, tomato, and red onion for garnish

**Directions:**

1. In a bowl, combine Greek yogurt, minced garlic, lemon juice, dried oregano, salt, and pepper.

2. Add the cubed chicken to the yogurt mixture and toss to coat. Marinate for 15-20 minutes.

3. Preheat a grill or grill pan to medium-high heat.

4. Thread the marinated chicken onto skewers.

5. Grill for 4-5 minutes per side until the chicken is cooked through and has grill marks.

6. Warm pita bread rounds on the grill for about 30 seconds on each side.

7. Serve chicken souvlaki in warmed pita bread, drizzled with tzatziki sauce, and garnished with sliced cucumber, tomato, and red onion.

**Nutritional Value (per serving):**

- Calories: 300

- Protein: 25g

- Carbohydrates: 30g

- Fiber: 3g

- Fat: 8g

**Recipe 47: Sweet Potato and Black Bean Tacos**

**Prep Time:** 30 minutes **Serves:** 4

**Ingredients:**

- 2 large sweet potatoes, peeled and diced

- 1 can (15 oz) black beans, drained and rinsed

- 1 teaspoon chili powder

- 1/2 teaspoon ground cumin

- Salt and pepper to taste

- 8 small whole-grain tortillas

- 1 cup shredded lettuce

- 1 cup diced tomatoes

- 1/2 cup diced red onion

- 1/2 cup fresh cilantro, chopped

- Juice of 2 limes

- Hot sauce for serving (optional)

**Directions:**

1. Preheat the oven to 425°F (220°C).

2. Toss diced sweet potatoes with olive oil, chili powder, ground cumin, salt, and pepper.

3. Spread sweet potatoes on a baking sheet and roast for 25-30 minutes until they are tender and slightly crispy.

4. In a large bowl, combine black beans, roasted sweet potatoes, and fresh cilantro.

5. In a separate bowl, mix diced tomatoes, diced red onion, lime juice, salt, and pepper.

6. Warm the tortillas in a dry skillet or microwave.

7. Assemble the tacos by placing the sweet potato and black bean mixture on each tortilla.

8. Top with shredded lettuce, tomato and onion salsa, and a drizzle of hot sauce if desired.

**Nutritional Value (per serving):**

- Calories: 250

- Protein: 8g

- Carbohydrates: 50g

- Fiber: 10g

- Fat: 2g

**Recipe 48: Mango and Avocado Salad**

**Prep Time:** 20 minutes **Serves:** 4

**Ingredients:**

- 2 ripe mangoes, peeled, pitted, and diced

- 2 ripe avocados, peeled, pitted, and diced

- 1/4 cup red onion, finely chopped

- 1/4 cup fresh cilantro, chopped

- Juice of 1 lime

- 1 tablespoon olive oil

- Salt and pepper to taste

**Directions:**

1. In a large bowl, combine diced mangoes, diced avocados, chopped red onion, and chopped cilantro.

2. Drizzle with lime juice and olive oil.

3. Season with salt and pepper.

4. Toss to combine all ingredients.

5. Serve immediately.

**Nutritional Value (per serving):**

- Calories: 250

- Protein: 2g

- Carbohydrates: 30g

- Fiber: 8g

- Fat: 15g

**Recipe 49: Broccoli and Cheddar Stuffed Potatoes**

**Prep Time:** 45 minutes **Serves:** 4

**Ingredients:**

- 4 large russet potatoes

- 2 cups broccoli florets, steamed and chopped

- 1 cup shredded cheddar cheese

- 1/2 cup Greek yogurt

- 2 tablespoons unsalted butter

- Salt and pepper to taste

- Chopped chives for garnish (optional)

## Directions:

1. Preheat the oven to 400°F (200°C).

2. Scrub and dry the russet potatoes. Prick them with a fork a few times.

3. Bake the potatoes directly on the oven rack for 45-60 minutes until they are tender when pierced with a fork.

4. While the potatoes bake, steam broccoli florets until tender. Chop them into small pieces.

5. When the potatoes are done, cut a slit lengthwise in the top of each potato.

6. Carefully scoop out the potato flesh, leaving a thin shell.

7. Mash the potato flesh with Greek yogurt, unsalted butter, shredded cheddar cheese, salt, and pepper.

8. Fold in the steamed and chopped broccoli.

9.  Stuff each potato shell with the broccoli and cheddar mixture.

10. Return the stuffed potatoes to the oven and bake for an additional 10-15 minutes until the cheese is melted and bubbly.

11. Garnish with chopped chives if desired.

**Nutritional Value (per serving):**

- Calories: 300

- Protein: 10g

- Carbohydrates: 45g

- Fiber: 6g

- Fat: 10g

**Recipe 50: Teriyaki Salmon**

**Prep Time:** 30 minutes **Serves:** 2

**Ingredients:**

- 2 salmon fillets

- 1/4 cup low-sodium soy sauce

- 2 tablespoons honey

- 1 tablespoon rice vinegar

- 1 clove garlic, minced

- 1 teaspoon fresh ginger, minced

- Sesame seeds and sliced green onions for garnish

- Steamed broccoli for serving (optional)

## Directions:

1. In a small bowl, whisk together low-sodium soy sauce, honey, rice vinegar, minced garlic, and minced ginger.

2. Place salmon fillets in a shallow dish and pour the teriyaki marinade over them.

3. Marinate the salmon for 15-20 minutes.

4. Preheat a grill or grill pan to medium-high heat.

5. Remove salmon from the marinade and grill for 4-5 minutes per side until the salmon is cooked through and has grill marks.

6. Garnish with sesame seeds and sliced green onions.

7. Serve with steamed broccoli if desired.

## Nutritional Value (per serving):

- Calories: 300

- Protein: 25g

- Carbohydrates: 20g

- Fiber: 1g

- Fat: 12g

# CONCLUSION

As we reach the end of "Breathing Easy: Nourishing Recipes for Asthma Wellness," we want to extend our heartfelt thanks for choosing this cookbook to guide your culinary journey. We hope that these asthma-friendly recipes have brought newfound joy to your kitchen and inspired you to prioritize your respiratory health through the meals you prepare.

Cooking is not merely a task; it is an art that allows us to nourish our bodies and souls. We firmly believe that with the right ingredients and mindful preparation, you can enjoy delicious and health-conscious dishes that support your asthma management.

Remember that asthma is just one facet of your life, and it should never define your experiences or limit your enjoyment of food. We encourage you to continue exploring the vast world of culinary delights, experimenting with flavors, and sharing meals with loved ones.

As you continue your journey toward better asthma wellness, remember that small changes in your diet can make a significant impact on your overall health. Stay curious, stay mindful, and savor the flavors of life with every bite.

We hope that "Breathing Easy" has not only enriched your recipe collection but also empowered you to embrace a lifestyle that prioritizes your well-being. By choosing asthma-friendly foods and adopting mindful cooking practices, you are taking proactive steps toward a healthier and more fulfilling life.

Thank you for joining us on this flavorful adventure, and may each meal you create be a testament to your dedication to a life filled with wellness and joy. Continue to breathe easy, savor the moments, and relish every culinary masterpiece you create.

Bon appétit, and here's to a future filled with good health and delicious dishes!